Back To Life

Emily

Copyright © 2018 Emily

All rights reserved.

ISBN: 9781981003624

CONTENTS

Acknowledgments

1	Introduction	1
2	Your Mind is Able to Relieve the Pain	3
3	The Checklist for a Healthy Back	29
4	Some Amazing Smoothies Recipes for Anti Inflammation	34

Readers are highly recommended to seek proper advice from either a physician or a professional practitioner before implementing any of these suggestions. Seriously, this book cannot replace professional and medical advice. Therefore, both the author and the publisher will not take any responsibility for any adverse results if readers really follow the information herein.

Introduction

Welcome to Back To Life. This incredible book will be suitable for anyone who is struggling with back pain, and who wants to look for the proper remedy. I know that more and more people are feeling stressed and losing hope right now. But don't give up so easily, because with this book, you can definitely find out the best solution to relieve your pain.

The movement introduced in this book aims to help you move your back and your entire body, which will create stability, as well as flexibility. Your spine will be supported and your back will become more limber. Therefore, you will be able to both sit and stand comfortably since these simple treatments will improve your posture. Also, applying the included breathing advice is very important too, as it will keep your muscles engaged efficiently and help you release the pressure on your back.

I am very excited for you to begin this journey. And on top of that, I am willing to hear your sharing and experience after following this amazing method and reviving your back!

-Emily

Your Mind is Able to Relieve the Pain

Your mind is one of the greatest things that your body has. If your body has had a pain for a long time, your mind tends to fixate on it. This situation is very normal, and you have to know it is one of the survival parts of your body. The pain affects our mind, so we usually have a thought to get away from it quickly. However, with back pain, things start to get worse. If your mind thinks about this pain, your muscles will have a tendency to tighten up, which will prevent the proper blood flow, then lead to aches and stiffness.

A long time ago, I learned to practice a very simple technique to relieve the pain. In particular, you will learn how to control where to put your attention. Therefore, instead of focusing on the painful parts of your body, you should think about the body parts which are pain-free intentionally. This intentional thought will help you to stop thinking about the painful aspects, and then start feeling better gradually. I have undertaken this technique many times and gotten very good results afterward.

De-stabilize your core

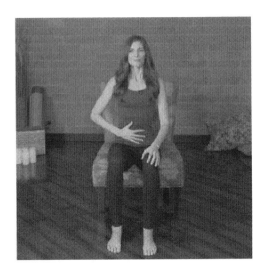

Prepare a chair and sit on the edge of your chair. Keep your posture nice and tall. Place your feet on the floor and place them the width of your hip. One of your two hands should be put on either your stomach or your belly button. Breathe deeply through your nose and when you exhale, you should feel your navel going down your spine, as well as go up your ribcage. When taking the next breath, you should hold your belly firmly.

The breath tends to expand widely into both your ribcage and your chest. However, you should not allow it to go down your abdomen. Keep your stomach tighter as you exhale and make it tight when inhaling.

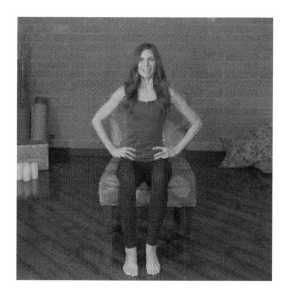

Then, put your hands at the front of your hip bones, you can feel the muscles of your lower abdomen through your fingertips. Try to exhale and think that you can use these abdominal muscles to make your hip bones go in towards one another. In fact, your hips will stay still, but you can feel the movement of the lower belly muscles. At this time, you need to relax your shoulders and fill up your chest and your ribcage with your breath. Always remember to keep your lower belly tight.

By breathing this way, you can feel the internal workings of your abdominal muscles. And of course, this is known as engaging or de-stabilizing your core. Do not forget to engage your core for the whole day. If you can engage your core muscles during your movement all day, you can practice your core with your simple daily movement without any barriers. There are a variety of daily activities for you to do and contract your core at the same time including:

- Slow running and walking
- Sitting on your desk
- Washing and drying your dishes

- Getting in and getting out of your car
- Getting up from a chair
- Bending down to tie the shoelaces
- Pick up the book on the floor
- Wearing your shirts or your pants

Simple core

During your exhale, I highly recommend that you should do the first out of three steps. Keep your position when inhaling. Then, you can do the following step for the next exhale. Continue to keep this position when inhaling. Finally, you can repeat for all three steps.

1. Make the lower belly go toward the spine
2. Imagine an elevator and make your belly button go up the ribcage
3. Let your hip bones go towards each other and squeeze tightly by making use of the lower abdominal muscles.

Exercise 1 for your core: Lift your knee

Firstly, you need to sit on a chair or the couch nice and tall. Place your hands on your hips with your fingertips toward the lower belly. Breathe deeply, and during your exhale, you need to draw your belly in and up. Next, you need to slightly tap your lower belly with your fingers. By doing this, you can dig into the muscles of your lower belly and wake them up. These muscles are placed in front of your hip crests and below your belly button.

Continue to inhale again while holding your belly tightly with your fingers. After that, exhale and lift your right knee by using your right lower abdominal muscles. And then, you can start lowering your right leg when you inhale and raise your left knee during your next exhale. This activity will contract your lower left abdominal muscles. But you should make sure to balance the weight on your hips when you lift the legs. Avoid leaning totally on only one side.

You can repeat these movements from the right to the left for a total of 10 times on each side.

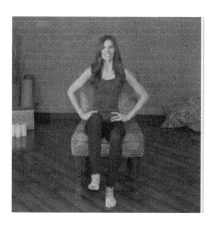 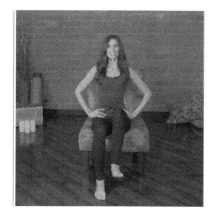

Tips to remember:

- Make sure your spine is tall. You cannot lean your back on anything when lifting your legs.
- For the most effective result, you should relax your shoulders since you do not need their support for this activity.
- Your abdominal muscles are playing an important role as the lever to raise your legs. And the way you exhale will increase the power for this lever.
- You can tuck your chin a little bit or make your jawline parallel with the floor. By this way, you can ensure that the back of your neck is long enough.

Exercise 2 for your core: Hold your knee

This exercise asks you to engage your core tightly while breathing in deeply. After that, try to raise your right knee as high as possible during your exhale. Do not lower your knee quickly. You should hold it up and take about 5 deep breaths. Make sure that you keep the weight balanced on both of your hips instead of putting all of the weight on your right hip. Also, you should keep the ribcage up from your hips and try to sit up tall. You can repeat these movements on your left side.

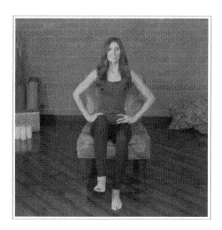 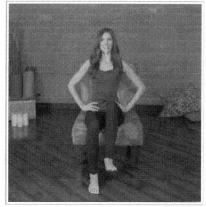

Tips to remember:
- Do not forget to take a full deep breath into your chest together with your ribs every time.
- During your exhale, you should tighten your stomach muscles as much as you can.
- Try to keep your forehead as well as your jaw relaxed.
- Make sure to sit up tall and strong.

Exercise 3 for your core: Twist your oblique

For this exercise, you can put your feet onto the floor at first. Remember to keep your feet at a hip's width apart and have a tall posture. Next, you can keep both of your hands behind your head. To have the correct position, your elbows need to be opened wide.

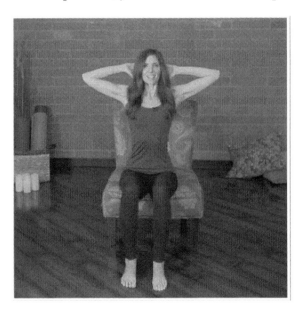

At this stage, breathe in deeply. Then, you can twist your body to the right when taking 3 pulsing exhales. When you renturn to the center, you need to inhale. Continue to twist to the left and take 4 pulsing exhales. You need to practice this exercise 10 rounds on each side.

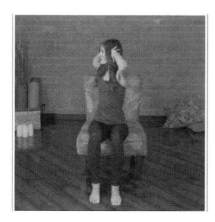 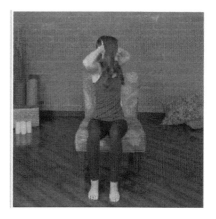

Every time you return to the center, make sure to sit up taller. Moreover, I highly advise that you should keep the length in your spine during your twist. And of course, you should draw your core muscles in tight. By this way, you can effectively wring out your abdominal muscles whenever you make a twist to the right or the left.

Tips to remember:

- Do not move your hips every time you twist. Also, your hips should be grounded firmly into the chair for the best result.
- Remember to relax your shoulders and do not raise them too much.
- Tuck your chin slightly to prevent you from looking up and hurting the back of your neck for each of your twists.

How to stretch and release your back: Forward Fold

Level 1

First of all, you need to place your feet a little farther in front of you. Then, you should bend your body forward slightly, which puts your chest totally onto your thighs. At this step, you can tuck your chin a little bit, which enables the back of your neck to relax the most. Now, your head's crown will hang toward the floor and your shoulders need to relax forward also.

Furthermore, you should pay attention and take some deep breaths. By this way, you can stretch your breaths into the muscles of your back. This activity will help you to feel comfortable and relaxed when making an exhale. You do not have to rush, you only need to breathe deeply and calmly. A good breath is considered as the key to release the tense and tight muscles in your body.

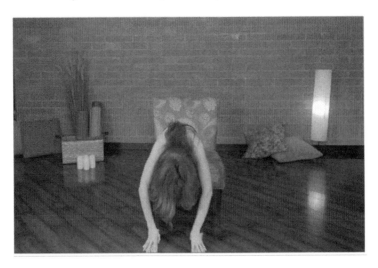

Level 2

For anyone who prefers a deeper stretch, you can go to level 2 by standing up and bending forward over your legs. Do not forget to have a real deep bend in your knees. Otherwise, you will strain your lower back, which is not a good sign for your health. With this level, it is very great if your hands can grab the elbows from the opposite side and hang your arms.

Your head needs to be hung also, and well, you should not attempt to either look up or look down at the ground.

Tips to remember:

- You can close your eyes to keep your body in the most relaxing condition.
- Use your nose to take a breath in and out, which will result in a good calming effect on many parts of your body.
- If you inhale and exhale correctly based on these instructions, you can get rid of the tension in your body efficiently.

Exercise for upper back: Goal post arms

Level 1: Upright Goal Post Arms

Again, I have to remind you to sit up on your chair tall and strong. Now, you need to keep your arms in the goal post position. In particular, both of your elbows should be raised and placed in line with your shoulders. If you have a correct posture, your elbows will create a 90-degree bend and your palms tend to face forward at the same time. Then, engage your core and try to exhale deeply to allow your shoulder blades to squeeze together on your back. At this time, your elbows, as well as your palms are going to draw back. However, you should remember to avoid arching your back forward too much. Now, you can release your elbows back to the original position and try your best to repeat this squeezing activity around 10 times.

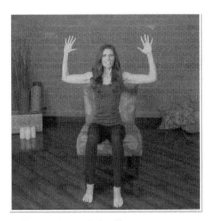 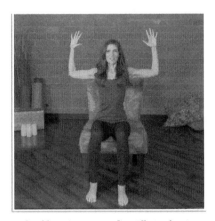

* Elbows in line with shoulders.   * Shoulders squeeze together. Elbows draw slightly back.

Level 2: Forward Bend Goal Post Arms

For level 2, you need to continue a goal post position for your arms. Then, you can lean your chest forward a little bit and hover them above your thighs. Make sure that your chin is tucked slightly to keep the back of your neck long and prevent it from being pinched. After that, you can squeeze your shoulder blades together, as well as raise the back of your arms toward the ceiling. Next, you can release your arms and keep them in the original posture. And then, you can repeat this process about 10 times before taking a break.

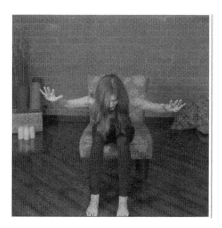
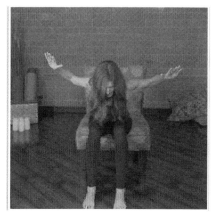

Tips to remember:

- Make sure that your shoulders are in line with your ears and do not let your chin jut forward.
- When you want to squeeze your shoulder blades together, you need to exhale. And of course, make sure to reverse this process if you want to release them.
- Your elbows, along with your palms, need to move in line with each other.

Exercise to relieve the neck and your shoulder: Stretch your chest

Level 1

You need to keep your arms behind you and clasp them together. Otherwise, you can grab your hands onto the back of your chair. Make sure that both of your shoulders are drawn back and down properly. Then, your chest needs to be raised and arched slightly forward. At this step, you can feel a real stretch not only in your chest, but also in front of your shoulders. Breathe deeply and allow the fresh air to fill up your chest when you inhale.

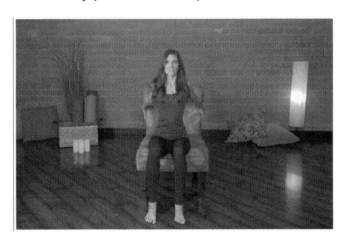

Level 2:

Moving to level 2, you need to find a doorway and make your arms into the goalpost posture by putting your albows and your hands onto the door frame. Your chest, together with your shoulder muscles, can gradually feel a bit of the stretch when you start leaning your chest forward. Use your nose to take a deep breath in and make the great attempt to hold this stretch in at least 30 seconds. If you do not feel comfortable, you can try lowering or lifting your elbows on the door frame according to your physical condition. Besides, you can try to change different angles for the best stretch.

Tips to remember:

- Do not forget to tuck your chin a little bit, so that the back of your neck will not become over-arched after your exercise.
- You can make use of your breath to practice stretching the muscles of your chest from the inside.

Exercise to support your low back: Glute strength

Level 1: Squeeze your glute or your buttock muscles

You are highly recommend to sit forward on your chair. Place your feet on the floor in front of you. Make sure that your feet are put a little bit farther apart than your knees. About your hands, you should place them on the chair and next to the position of your hips. Your core needs to be engaged and try to sit up tall. When you make the first exhale, you need to squeeze the glutes underneath you. You can feel that your hips are lifted a bit during your squeezing process. After that, you can release your glutes by inhaling. Remember to exhale when you squeeze and inhale when you release. If you reverse these process, it will create a lot of troubles. And for sure, you can repeat this squeezing motion about 20 times in total.

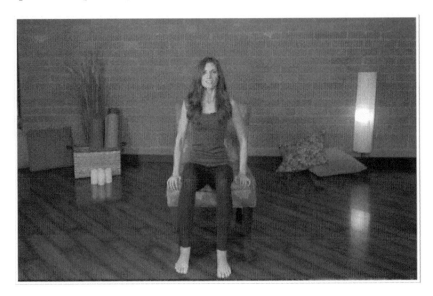

Level 2: Stand and sit

You need to place your hips farther back on your chair, but do not rest your back on the chair. In addition, your toes should be put a little apart and your feet should be placed wider than your hips width. Now, put your arms straight in front of your face and try to reach them forward. When doing this, you can breathe in deeply. Then, take a breath out to press into your heels and stand up at the same time. Simultaneously, you should squeeze your glutes and move your hips forward when you gradually stand up. Next, you can inhale and put your hips back to the chair. However, you should try hovering your hips over the chair a bit instead of actually touching the chair. After that, you can take a deep breath out again and stand up. Make sure to do this process again and again with 10 rounds.

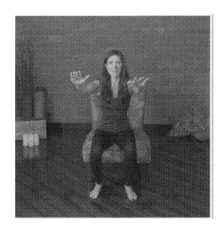 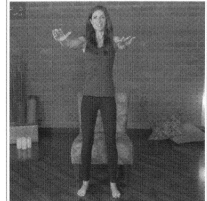

Tips to remember:
- You cannot let both of your knees to either lean, collapse or touch each other. You have to keep them look at the same point as your toes.
- Do not rush since you can perform these moevements slowly and in a controlled motion.

Stretch your hip and your glute: Seated Pigeon Stretch (which can eliminate the Sciatica)

For the first step, you are highly advised to sit up tall on the chair and then roll two sides of your shoulders onto your back. Then, you can put your feet on the ground at a hips width apart and notice if your knees are bent at 90 degrees. Next, you should cross your right ankle over your left thigh and make sure to flex your right foot. By this way, you can balance the joint of your right knee. After that, do not forget to gently press your right hand onto your right knee and toward the floor. When doing this movement, you have to feel the stretch on your right hip, as well as your right buttock muscle. In case you do not feel the stretch, you need to stop a bit and try to reach your chest forward. Repeat the pressing and continue to expand your chest until you can feel the stretch. You need to keep this stretch up to 30 seconds while breathing deeply. After finishing with one side, you can repeat this process with the other side.

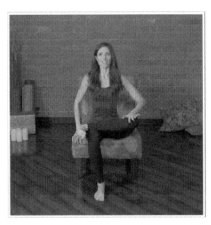 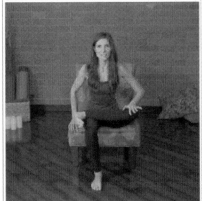

Tips to remember:
- This exercise is very suitable for those people who are struggling with sciatica and lower back pain. You should

attempt to do this movement at least 3 times daily. In case you might forget, you should remind yourself by putting post-it notes onto your working place or setting the reminder on your mobile phone.

- You can apply this stretch on your back by crossing your right ankle over your left knee. And then, your left knee should be drawn into your chest.

Exercise to support your low back: Stretch your hip flexor

This exercise aims to turn your body to the left and then scoot your hip to the front edge of your chair. You can use your left hand to hold the back of your chair. Then, put your left hip on the chair and move your right knee to touch down the floor. With this posture, you can totally feel the stretch on your right hip and your right thigh. Keep this position for 30 seconds and do not forget to take a deep breath in. Repeat this process with the other side.

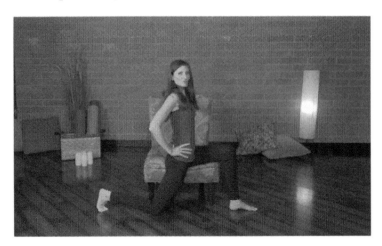

Tips to remember:
- The front of your hip of the leg that you kneel down has to feel the stretch. Otherwise, you need to press your hip forward more until you can feel the real stretch.
- For those people who tend to sit a lot, you may suffer from the tight hip flexors. As a result, trying to stretch out these parts will align your pelvic as well as your spine better.

- If you want to challenge yourself, you can do this stretch while standing up by simply grabbing the back of your chair. At this moment, you can keep your balance with your left leg. Next, try to hold the top of your right foot behind your hips after bending your right knee. Right now, your knee should be drawn back as you press your hip to the front. It is better if you can remove your hands from the chair and keep the balance.

Exercise to flex and extend your spine: Seated cat cows

Try to sit forward and put your hands on both of your knees. You should take a deep breath in and make sure your shoulders are drawn in together when arching your chest to the front, as well as raising your chin a little bit. Then, you can slowly take your breath out and draw your skin toward your chest while rounding your back to the back of the chair. When you breathe in, remember to arch your chest forward. On the other hand, when breathing out, it is time to round back. No need to hurry since you are suggested to do this calmly. You should notice your back to exactly know how far you can bend. It will create good results if you can repeat this exercise 10 times.

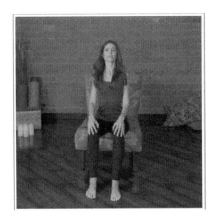 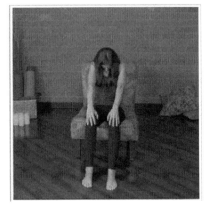

Tips to remember:
- When you take a breath in and raise your chest at the same time, make sure that your neck does not bend back too much. Instead of your neck bending, you should focus on the length of the front of your throat.
- Your core needs to be slightly engaged to allow your lower back to stabilize better.

Exercise to stretch your lateral: Bend your sides

First and foremost, you should try to reach your right hand to touch the outer part of your left thigh. And of course, you need to stretch your left hand up in the air. With this stretch, you can feel that your ribcage is being lifted, as well as your spine is growing more.

Keep this posture and take a breath out. You can try to reach your arm over your head and bend it to the opposite side. At this step, your left hip will be pressed down to the chair, therefore, your left fingers need to reach farther. I highly recoomend that you should inhale deeply 3 to 5 times to fill up your left ribcage. After that, start inhaling to get back to the center and repeat this process on the opposite side.

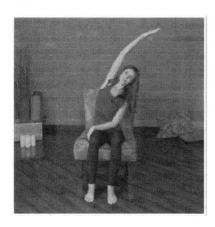 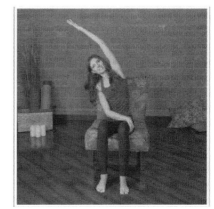

Tips to remember:
- If you breathe deeply, you will be able to stretch the intercostal muscle of your ribcage better and longer.
- Make sure that you do not hunch your chest forward. Moreover, your shoulders should be squared forward.

Exercise to rotate your spine: Seated twist

You need to put your right hand on the outer side of your left thigh. Then, place your left hand on the back of the chair behind your back. At the same time, you need to turn your chin and look over your right shoulder. After that, take a deep breath in and keep your posture. Next, take a breath out and try to make a deeper twist than the previous one. You can use your hands to support your spine during this twist. And especially, you should keep this twist for 3 to 5 breaths. After these breaths, you can get back to the center and take a little break. After the break, you can repeat the whole process on the opposite side.

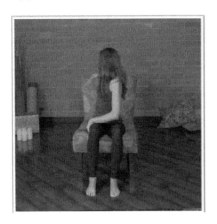 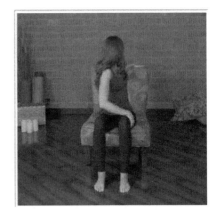

Tips to remember:

Remember to keep your posture tall enough. And make sure that your spine does not round back even once.

Exercise to stretch your neck

This exercise requires you to reach your left arm to the side to form a half 'A'. This will draw a line from your ear to your left shoulder. At the same time, your right ear tends to lower down a little bit towards your shoulder. It will look like you are keeping something between your ear and your shoulder. Inhale deeply and your shoulders will melt down more every time you make an exhale.

Keep your posture for 3 to 5 deep breaths.

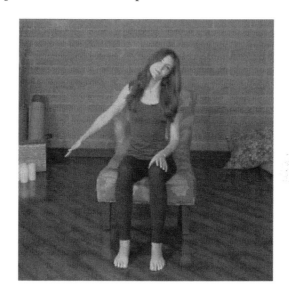

It is time to keep your chin down, and it looks like you are looking down onto your right-side pocket. Raise your left arm slightly in order to help you feel the stretch more clearly. Especially, you can feel the stretch from your neck, as well as in the front of your chest. Continue to hold this position for 3 to 5 times when you breathe.

Do not forget to perform this movement on both sides before taking a break.

Last but not least, lowering and releasing your left arm and make sure to tuck your chin forward to your chest. Take a deep breath to be able to strech out the back of your neck correctly. Again, keep this position for 3 to 5 deep breaths.

Now, you can raise your head and looking straight. You can feel relieved and release all of your pressure in your body.

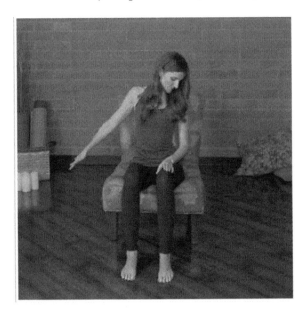

Tips to remember:
- Your chest should be always raised properly and make sure that your shoulders do not cave forward too much.
- Do not put much pressure on your neck when doing these stretches. This part needs to be in the most relaxing condition. And well, you can let the gravity draw your head's direction.

The Checklist for a Healthy Back

Welcome back to the checklist for your healthy back. This wonderful checklist will give you a number of incredible tips and methods that you can apply every day. By following them, not only your back but also your overall health will be improved significantly.

With my experience, these tricks are very simple and easy to follow. However, the hardest part for most of us is to remember them clearly and correctly. As a consequence, you should not try to complete all of them throughout your day. Instead, you can choose some tips that are the most suitable for yourself and make them into your habit. Furthermore, you can set the reminders on your phone, as well as write some notes and stick them onto the fridge.

Align your posture

- Try to split the weight evenly on your feet instead of leaning the whole weight to only one side. Make sure to set both of your feet under your hip sockets. Also, your toes should be turned to the front.
- Remember to cave your ankles outward properly. Moreover, you can roll some weight onto the outside edges of your feet. By this way, you can raise your arches slightly and keep your ankles as stable as possible. At the same time, your knees will be able to knock outward appropriately.
- Your knees should not be locked, instead, let them bend subtly and comfortably.
- Make sure that both sides of your hips can be in the neutral position. Furthermore, they are capable of squeezing your glutes gently so as to improve your lower back.
- Do not forget to make your navel go inward and upward repeatedly to de-stabilize your core. By this way, your lower back will be brought back to the nertral position and avoid swaying forward.
- You should limit any activities that can hurt your lower or middle back. Therefore, you should put your shoulder blades together if it does not hurt your back. Thanks to this motion, you can have a nice feeling for your chest as well as your upper back.
- Turn your chin back a little bit to make your ears stay right over your shoulders.

When you sit

- You are highly advised to put your feet on the floor instead of crossing your legs. In case your feet cannot reach the floor, you might need the put some books or a stool under your feet.

- Your shoulders should be relaxed, and you can try to squeeze them together frequently. By this way, you can avoid the rounding issue for your upper back.
- You should not lean your chin to the front. Rather than doing that, you should lift your ears over your shoulders. The reason is that your neck muscles have to get strained more when your chin is leaned forward.

At your desk

- Trying to lift your laptop screen to make it suitable for your eye level.
- Sit on the chair with a tall and strong posture. As you type, your elbows need to be placed next to your ribs. Some people usually keep them reach forward with their arms, which is not a right posture.
- For every hour, you should get up and walk around for a while. I notice that keeping your body moving is very important.
- If your work requires using the mobile phone all the time, you need to prepare a headset. Keeping your phone in the middle of your ear and your shoulder is not a good point.
- Make sure to look at your mobile phone at your eye level whenever you are texting or when you are on the Internet. Always looking down on your phone will make your neck strain too much. You may hear the word 'Text Neck', which is a common issue for people nowadays.

Make your load lighter and balanced

Carrying heavy bags and backpacks on a regular basis will do harm to your back. If you really have to carry a bag, remember that you have to switch the bags between both hands frequently. When you always carry the bag with only one arm, you are creating the imbalance for your body and especially your back.

Maintain the right sleeping position

- Many people have a habit of sleeping on their sides. If you are among these people, you should have a pillow between your knees. Make sure that the pillow is suitable for your height so that it can go in between both your knees and your ankles. I recommend using the body pillow, which is designed perfectly for your whole body. Thus, you can place your arms on it as well.
- For those people who are sleeping on their backs, you should place a pillow on the back of your knees.
- I do not encourage you to sleep on your stomach.

Release your stress

- You can breathe deeply and calmly with your nose. Whenever you make an exhale, you should think that your breath will remove all of your stress by carrying it outside your body. Then, you can feel that your shoulder mucles, as well as your neck muscles start melting. If you breathe in the right way, only a few breaths will make you feel better instantly.
- Try to walk around. Changing your vision is a great way to reduce your stress. As a result, you should take a walk in only 5 minutes and move your body comfortably while breathing the fresh air.
- Get the chance to change your mind. Every time you feel frustrated, tired and full of pessimism in your head, you should change your mind by practicing having the optimistic thoughts. For instance, you can talk to yourself that 'Everything happens for a reason' or 'Tommorrow will be better for sure'. I am sure that you will not totally believe in your words, but practicing these positive thoughts gradually will make you feel more and more relieved.

Choose the right shoes

Wearing shoes that are a smaller or larger size will affect your back, but many people do not notice. Moreover, you should not frequently wear high heels since it does not support your arch. I highly advise choosing shoes that are good for your arch and this should be on your priority list.

Pay attention while walking

If you accidentally fall while walking, it will have a negative impact on your back and also your body. Therefore, you should focus on everything around you during your walk.

Drive carefully

You may know that driving carefully will help you reduce the chance of car accidents, which will damage your back severely. You should be always cautious and stop texting while driving. Protecting yourself on the road is the same as protecting your health.

Enhance your balance

Balance is the vital factor that prevents you from tripping. Therefore, having great balance will support your core strength. Trying to practice your balance every day by standing on one foot is a great suggestion.

Plan your diet and have good nutrition

- Drink water as much as possible.
- Avoid food that causes inflamation.
- Avoid smoking.
- Limit your alcohol consumption.

Some Amazing Smoothies Recipes for Anti Inflammation

Are you looking for smoothies recipes which are perfect to improve your energy and burn your calories? If yes, these following recipes make you satisfied and happy after drinking them.

Protein Green Smoothie

Ingredients:

- ¼ cup organic Greek yogurt

- ½ cup almond milk

- 1/8 teaspoon spirulina

- ¼ cup cucumber

- ½ cup spinach

- 1 cup parsley

- ¼ cup fresh or frozen peaches

- ½ banana

- 2 teaspoons hemp seeds

- ½ cup ice

Directions:

Put all of these ingredients into the blender. Start blending until it is smooth.

Coconut Protein Green Smoothie

Ingredients:

- ½ cup coconut milk

- ½ cup coconut yogurt

- 2 teaspoons hemp seeds

- 1 teaspoon chia seeds

- 1 cup spinach

- 1 cup raw kale

- 1 green apple

- 1 teaspoon raw honey

- 1 teaspoon bee pollen

- ½ cup ice

Directions:

Put all of these ingredients into the blender. Start blending until it

gets smooth.

Coconut Blueberry Protein Smoothie

Ingredients:

- ½ cup Greek yogurt

- ½ cup coconut water

- ¼ cup blueberries

- ¼ cup fresh or frozen coconut

- 1 teaspoon bee pollen

- 1 teaspoon honey

- ½ cup ice

Directions:

put all of these ingredients into the blender. Start blending until it gets smooth.

Strawberry Flax Smoothie

Ingredients:

- ¼ cup coconut milk

- ¼ cup Greek yogurt

- ½ cup spinach

- 1 cup frozen strawberries

- ½ cup fresh pineapple

- 1 tablespoon ground flaxseeds

- 1 teaspoon honey

- ½ cup ice

Directions:

Put all of these ingredients into the blender. Start blending until it gets smooth.

Almond Berry Smoothie

Ingredients:

- ½ cup coconut water

- ¼ cup Greek yogurt

- 2 tablespoons almond butter

- ¼ cup blueberries

- ¼ cup raspberries

- ½ cup spinach

- ½ banana

- 1 tablespoon ground flaxseeds

- 1 tablespoon hemp seeds

- 1 tablespoon chia seeds

- ½ cup ice

Directions:

Put all of these ingredients into the blender. Start blending until it

gets smooth.

Oat Berry Protein Smoothie

Ingredients:

- ½ cup almond milk

- ½ cup Greek yogurt

- 2 tablespoons oats

- ¼ cup berries

- ½ cup spinach

- ½ banana

- 1 tablespoon ground flaxseeds

- 1 tablespoon hemp seeds

- ½ cup ice

Directions:

Put all of these ingredients into the blender. Start blending until it gets smooth.

Pumpkin Seed Oat Smoothie

Ingredients:

- ½ cup almond milk

- ¼ cup Greek yogurt

- 2 tablespoons oats

- ¼ cup raspberries

- 2 tablespoons pumpkin seeds

- 1 tablespoon ground flaxseeds

- 1 tablespoon hemp seeds

- 1 tablespoon chia seeds

- ½ cup ice

Directions:

Combine all ingredients in a blender. Blend until smooth.

High Protein Fig Smoothie

Ingredients:

- ½ cup coconut water

- ½ cup Greek yogurt

- 2 fresh figs

- ½ cup fresh or frozen strawberries

- ½ banana

- 1 teaspoon ground flaxseeds

- 1 teaspoon honey

- ½ cup ice

Directions:

Put all of these ingredients into the blender. Start blending until it

gets smooth.

Pineapple Ginger Smoothie

Ingredients:

- ½ cup almond milk

- ¼ cup Greek yogurt

- ½ cup raw kale

- 1 cup fresh or frozen pineapple

- 1 teaspoon honey or agave nectar

- ½ teaspoon of fresh ginger, grated

- 1 tablespoon lemon juice

- ½ cup ice

Directions:

Put all of these ingredients into the blender. Start blending until it gets smooth.

Mango Ginger Smoothie

Ingredients:

- ½ cup coconut milk

- ¼ cup Greek yogurt

- ½ cup raw kale

- ½ cup mango

- ½ orange

- 1 teaspoon agave nectar

- ½ teaspoon of fresh ginger, grated

- ½ cup ice

Directions:

Combine all ingredients in a blender. Blend until smooth.

Blueberry Bee Pollen Smoothie

Ingredients:

- ½ cup almond milk

- ¼ Greek yogurt

- ½ teaspoon bee pollen

- ½ banana

- ½ cup frozen blueberries

- ½ cup ice

Directions:

Put all of these ingredients into the blender. Start blending until it gets smooth.

Green Protein Smoothie

Ingredients:

- ½ cup coconut water

- ¼ cup Greek yogurt

- ½ cup raw kale

- 1 cucumber

- 1 cup fresh or frozen green grapes

- 1 banana

- 1 teaspoon ground flaxseeds

- ¼ teaspoon spirulina

- ½ cup ice

Directions:

Put all of these ingredients into the blender. Start blending until it gets smooth.

Berry Blast Smoothie

Ingredients:

- ½ cup almond milk

- ¼ cup Greek yogurt

- ½ teaspoon bee pollen

- ½ banana

- ½ cup frozen berries

- 1 cup fresh pineapple

- 1 teaspoon ground flaxseeds

- ½ cup ice

Back To Life

Directions:

Put all of these ingredients into the blender. Start blending until it gets bsmooth.

Berry Chia Smoothie

Ingredients:

- ½ cup coconut water

- ¼ cup Greek yogurt

- ½ cup frozen berries

- ½ cucumber

- 1 tablespoon ground chia seeds

- 1 teaspoon honey

- ½ cup ice

Directions:

Put all of these ingredients into the blender. Start blending until it gets smooth.

Chia Green Smoothie

Ingredients:

- ½ cup coconut water

- ¼ cup Greek yogurt

- ½ cup parsley

- 1 cup kale leaves

- ½ cucumber

- ¼ cup pineapple

- 1 tablespoon chia seeds

- ½ cup ice

Directions:

Put all of these ingredients into the blender. Start blending until it gets smooth.

Avocado Protein Smoothie

Ingredients:

- ½ cup coconut water

- ¼ cup Greek yogurt

- ½ cup raw kale

- ½ cup kiwi

- 1/2 avocado

- 2 tablespoons hemp seeds

- 1 teaspoon honey or agave

- ½ cup ice

Directions:

Put all of these ingredients into the blender. Start blending until it gets smooth.

Kefir Protein Berry Smoothie

Ingredients:

- 1 cup plain kefir

- ½ cup mixed fresh or frozen berries

- 1 apple

- ½ banana

- 2 tablespoons hemp seeds

- 1 teaspoon chia seeds

- ½ cup ice

Directions:

Put all of these ingredients into the blender. Start blending until it gets smooth.

Kefir Protein Green Smoothie

Ingredients:

- 1 cup plain kefir

- ½ cup kale

- ½ teaspoon spirulina

- 1 orange

- 2 tablespoons hemp seeds

- 1 teaspoon chia seeds

- ½ cup ice

Directions:

Put all of these ingredients into the blender. Start blending until it gets smooth.

Kefir Super Protein Smoothie

Ingredients:

- 1 cup plain kefir

- ¼ Greek yogurt

- ½ cup fresh or frozen mango

- ½ cucumber

- ½ green apple

- 1 tablespoon oats

- 2 tablespoons hemp seeds

- 1 teaspoon chia seeds

- ½ cup ice

Directions:

Put all of these ingredients into the blender. Start blending until it gets smooth.

Back To Life

Peanut Butter Berry Smoothie

Ingredients:
- ½ cup plain Greek yogurt

- ½ cup coconut water

- 1 ½ tablespoon peanut butter

- ½ cup mixed fresh or frozen berries

- ½ banana

- 1 tablespoon honey

- ½ cup ice

Directions:
Putall of these ingredients into the blender. Start blending until it gets smooth.

Green Almond Smoothie

Ingredients:
- ½ cup plain Greek yogurt

- ½ cup almond milk

- 1 ½ tablespoon almond butter

- 1 tablespoon oats

- ½ cup kale

- ¼ cup parsley

- ½ banana

- 1 tablespoon honey

- ½ cup ice

Directions:

Put all of these ingredients into the blender. Start blending until it gets smooth.

Printed in Great Britain
by Amazon